Fitness Nutrition

Top 20 Nutrition Tips to Get in Shape

By
Bring on Fitness

information contained within this document, including, but not limited to, errors, omissions, or inaccuracies.

About Bring On Fitness

Our passion for fitness gave life to **Bring On Fitness**. We started with the goal of helping as many people as we can. To educate, motivate and to help change peoples lives for the better. Bring On Fitness is not only for the fitness enthusiasts, but also for the beginner. We strongly believe nothing is more important than learning the basics and creating a strong foundation in both nutrition - through meal planning, and in exercise - by following a specific plan. This is just as important for the beginner, as it is for the experienced athlete.

We set high standards for ourselves, the information we share, and the products we carry. Our goal is to provide you with exceptional products that suit your needs and the knowledge and motivation to help you work towards and achieve your health and fitness goals.

Check us out at www.bringonfitness.com

"Our Mission is to have a positive impact in changing peoples lives. We will deliver the best possible fitness and nutrition solutions that will empower people to achieve their health and fitness goals."

Table of Contents

Introduction

I want to thank you for choosing this book, *"Fitness Nutrition: Top 20 Nutrition Tips to Get in Shape."*

You probably think that getting in shape requires you to spend hours at the gym and deprive yourself of food. Most people are programmed to believe that they have to treat their bodies harshly so they can get in shape. You want to drop the excess pounds, but you dread the thought of having to go through that supposedly painful ordeal, but what if you could lose weight as easily and as safely as possible without having to torture yourself? Is it possible? Of course, it is. All it requires is some discipline and a bit of patience on your part.

In fact, if you are determined and follow all the tips given in this book, you will never have to worry about fitting into your old clothes again. In this book, you will find 20 nutritional tips that are extremely easy to follow.

You probably have had enough of those preachy books that offer you some redundant content, aside from unrealistic diet plans. This book focuses more on getting enough nutrition out of food rather than weight loss. Proper nutrition is the key to a healthy body and mind. Weight loss certainly follows, but it is a by-product of eating healthy instead of having to starve yourself.

The language used throughout the book is simple, and each tip is explained in detail. This book contains all the possible information you would ever need as far as nutritional tips are concerned. From how to make a grocery list to how much water you should drink every day, this book has it all.

I sincerely hope that you enjoy reading this book, following all the tips, getting in shape, and staying that way.

20 Nutrition Tips to Get in Shape

The adage "**You are what you eat**" is true to a large extent. Time and again, it has been proven that a good nutritious diet is what leads to a healthy body.

Food contains six different types of nutrients that include macronutrients (fats, proteins and carbs), micronutrients (minerals and vitamins), and water. If this combination is interrupted, it becomes difficult for the body to function properly, and it becomes hard for you to accomplish your weight loss goals. Good nutrition provides energy and protects you from all types of chronic illnesses. Combine it with regular physical activity, and you can maintain a steady weight for as long as you live.

It is important to know how to make optimum use of nutrition and make it an essential part of your lifestyle. Let's have a look at some nutrition tips, which can help you lead a healthy lifestyle while shedding that excess weight.

Tip #1: Create a Grocery List

If you are serious about staying in shape, your days of carefree grocery shopping need to end. No more picking unhealthy, processed items or stocking up on any sugary drinks. You need to enter the supermarket with a carefully prepared list of foods you plan to buy. Take some time out during the weekend, and write down all the items that you will need to buy for the entire week.

Creating a shopping list, especially when you are eating clean, may seem easy to some but baffling to others. If you don't know where to start, let us help you organize your shopping list.

Below are the different approaches to making a shopping list:

The perpetual list:

This applies to the list of add-on items in your fridge. Foods that might need a re-fill or replacement may include honey, cooking wine, vinegar, etc.

The categorical list:

You can segregate the foods into different categories based on which section of the supermarket they are found. Then, carefully arrange the categories once again based on how you plan to traverse the store. That way, you won't be running back and forth trying to get the items you have missed and, as a result, will save time.

The recurring list:

List down all the food that you may want to buy every week; print an extra copy, and stick it on the fridge door.

The geographical list:

If you are a visual thinker, you can map out a floor plan of the store. Later, the foods can be added based on where they are located in the store.

Tip #2: Shop the Perimeter of the Grocery Store

Typically, the healthiest foods reside at the back or the outer sides of the grocery store. Often, these are the foods that contain the most nutrition and the least preservatives. While shopping, you should always ask yourself whether what you are buying is healthy or not. For these reasons, it's important to read the labels and simply glance through the ingredients.

The smartest way to go about picking the right foods is to look for fewer ingredients. The lower the number, the healthier the pick. If you see more than five ingredients on the label, you might want to put that packet down and look for something better. Most foods that are being sold on the outer isle (perimeter) are healthy, contain less sugar, have lower fat content, and are free of chemicals. These are food you should be picking.

Tip #3: Calculate Your Calorie Intake

As a general rule, if you consume more calories than you burn, you are bound to gain weight. Train yourself to count your calories per meal without going crazy over it. The trick is to be conscious of how many calories you are ingesting only for a week or so. As the days go by, you will automatically be programmed to consuming only a limited amount of calories.

Ensure that you work out every day for at least 45 minutes to burn the calories you ingested. Aside from your calorie intake, your stress levels, activity levels, sleep schedule, and hormonal levels all play a part in helping you get closer to your desired weight loss goals.

Tip #4: Clean your Cupboard

Even if you have been planning to eat healthily for a while, chances are that your cupboard is still packed with junk, and we don't only mean potato chips. The hidden sugars, sodium, or preservatives in your energy bars or pretzels are equally harmful to your health. Most of these products aren't any better than a candy bar.

Read the labels at the back of the product, and clear them off your shelf if they contain anything unhealthy. Replace them with air-popped popcorn (3 cups of popcorn contain no more than 100 calories) or some roasted nuts. You can pick all your favorite munchies as long as they provide nutrition and amount to less than 100 calories.

Another food item that you need to stay away from is high-sugar cereal. Bear in mind that even the supposedly healthy choices, such as gluten-free products and granola, also come under this category.

You can load up on lots of whole grain products, such as quinoa, wheat noodles, and brown rice. Low-sodium beans can provide you with much-needed fiber and protein, while cans of sardines and tuna can give you omega-3s.

Tip #5: Include Whole Foods, and cut down on Processed Foods

We understand. Making dietary changes is not easy. A trip to the grocery store can instantly turn into a minefield. There are all sorts of unhealthy but tempting food items just waiting for you to pick them. You may start with the organic section but unknowingly find yourself making way to the processed food section, and bam! Within minutes, your cart is overflowing with processed foods and sugary drinks.

There are also social gatherings where you typically end up eating a sinful spread just to fit in. So how exactly do you make the transition? The key is to start replacing processed items in your kitchen with whole foods, one by one. Replace the white bread with brown bread, and use whole wheat flour for baking. Instead of sipping on sugary drinks, you can make your lemonade using honey, or eat a light meal before you head out to a party. The trick is to take it slowly and not make any sudden changes that you can't stick to. Additionally, you can follow the tips mentioned below that can help you adapt to a healthier lifestyle easily.

- Read the labels carefully before buying. Look for the amount of sugar, sodium, or fat percentage present in the product, and then make a choice.
- Take your own snacks to the office or even parties.

- Keep your kitchen shelves stocked with all kinds of fresh fruit and veggies to ensure you munch on healthy food items.

Tip #6: Weekly Meal Prep

If you feel overwhelmed at the thought of meal prep, take a minute to look at it differently. Prepping for your meals does not always have to be a tedious task. If anything, it will make your life much easier. All you have to do is take some time out to come up with easy ideas that can save you time and money.

Sunday meal preps can be fun if you involve your partner or even your kids in the process. Planning your weekly meals on a Sunday helps you kick-start your week with a healthy and fresh mindset. If you plan to do grocery shopping on Saturday, you can simply organize all the food items the next day. Make a list of your daily meals for the entire week from Monday through Friday. You might want to eat some turkey on Monday, ham on Tuesday, pork tenderloin on Wednesday, and so on. There are multiple benefits to meal prepping, and some of them are listed below.

- Saves you time and money

- Less cheating

- Greater variety

- Stress-free routine

Tip #7: Pick the Right Meal Plan

It's no secret that eating clean is the key to staying lean. Once you have decided to clear your kitchen of all unhealthy products, you can focus on picking the right meal plan.

There is no such thing as one perfect meal plan that works for everyone. Depending on your nutritional requirements, you might need different diet plans. A healthy meal should include the right amount of proteins (nuts, eggs, fish, meat, beans, and dairy), simple carbohydrates, and lots of fiber (fruits, whole-grains & vegetables). Following a customized meal plan will not only help you stay in shape but will also meet your nutritional needs. So how exactly does one create perfect meals? Below are some steps that may help you.

- Find out where exactly you stand compared to where you want to be when it comes to consuming the right foods. Do you need to cut down on your carb intake or increase your protein consumption?
- Work out as much as you eat. Keeping track of your calorie deficit will help you stay focused on your goal.
- Eat your macros. Check if you are eating the right amount of proteins, fats, and carbohydrates.
- Consider using fitness apps like MYFITNESS PAL to customize your macros and calories.

Tip #8: Eat Protein with Every Meal

The world is so protein-obsessed today that it's tricky to figure out how much of it you need to get in shape. This depends on your age, sex, activity level, and whether you are breastfeeding or pregnant. However, in general, you need about 1 gram of protein per pound of your actual body weight. Some of the rich sources of protein are yogurt, eggs, meat, and poultry. Although typically, proteins come from your regular meals, a lot of people prefer to take protein shakes. Unless you are following an intense workout regime, you don't need to rely on external protein supplements.

Tip #9: Don't Skip Your Breakfast

The fact that a lot of people consider breakfast to be the most important meal of the day may be debatable. However, based on studies, people who regularly eat breakfast tend to be healthier than those who don't.

Although skipping breakfast alone cannot make you gain weight, it does help you eat healthier and feel more energetic throughout the day. Eating your breakfast on time also means that you won't be overeating at lunch time. You may think that eliminating breakfast can reduce your overall calorie intake, but skipping it can make you feel lethargic, grumpy and less motivated to carry on with your day. A protein- and fiber-rich breakfast can prove to be extremely beneficial for those who are trying to stay in shape. Certain studies have also shown that consuming breakfast can also boost your metabolism. A few things you should keep in mind as regards breakfast are as follows:

- Breakfast doesn't always have to be a heavy meal. It can also mean eating a bowl of fruit, egg whites, or a portion of oatmeal and fresh yogurt.

- Morning meals can also have a positive effect on the blood sugar concentration in your body.

- Training on an empty stomach does work in your favor, but don't forget to eat your breakfast immediately after the workout.

Tip #10: Drink One Glass of Water before each Meal

If there was one super simple technique to lose weight, enhance your skin, and keep yourself energetic, that would be to drink as much water as you can throughout the day. It doesn't cost a thing. Keeping yourself hydrated at all times can work like magic when it comes to your overall health. Drinking one glass of water before every meal can also reap huge benefits. The most important ones are listed below.

Weight loss

Several studies have proven that gulping down some water before every meal can help you to consume fewer calories, and this will eventually result in weight loss. This can also be because water may leave you feeling fuller, and you may not need as much food to feel satisfied. That being said, ensure that you drink water at least 20 minutes before having your meals.

Improves skin

Drinking water before every meal is not going to suddenly cut years off the look of your skin, but it will certainly help in hydrating dry skin, especially during winter. You may not feel like drinking enough water during winter, and this can make you feel itchy and lifeless. Drinking enough water before and after your meals is vital, regardless of the weather.

Keeps you energetic

Have you ever noticed a major drop in your energy levels, only to realize that you haven't had enough water? You need an ample amount of water for your body's internal systems to function smoothly, and if you are already feeling thirsty, chances are that by the time you realize this, you are already dehydrated. You can avoid this by simply drinking water at regular intervals, especially before your meals.

Tip #11: Limit Meal Variety

Diets are created with the aim of limiting your food consumption, but people often overeat assuming that eating healthy food is never going to make them gain weight. That's not true. If you take in more calories than you burn, regardless of how healthy your diet is, you are bound to gain weight.

The trick is to watch your portion size, and track your calories with every meal. However, if you are a foodie like me who can't seem to control your taste buds, limiting your meal variety can help. The fact that "variety" in meals causes you to overeat is based on the concept of "sensory fullness or satiety." It is centered on a specific theory that states that the first bite of food is always the most satisfying, and subsequently, the pleasure diminishes. So when you have too much meal variety to choose from, first bites could mean too many calories consumed. That's exactly what happens at buffets. Variety doesn't necessarily have to lead to weight gain, but you will certainly find it easier to control your portion sizes when the spread is limited.

Tip #12: Pick Lean Proteins

We assume that meat is the best source of protein. It is assumed that as long as you are enjoying your steak, you are consuming enough proteins. However, some of these packed meats are also linked to some serious illnesses, such as certain cancers and heart diseases.

It is imperative that you pick lean and unprocessed proteins for your daily diet. One of the best ways to achieve your desired weight loss goals is to include lots of lean proteins in your diet.

Consuming lean protein helps you maintain healthy cholesterol levels while reducing the risk of life-threatening illnesses or heart disease. According to the Mayo Clinic, lean protein contains not more than 3 grams of fat and about 50 calories per serving. The clinic also recommends 46 grams of a daily dose of protein for women and 56 grams for men. Some of the best sources of lean protein can be found in the foods mentioned below.

- Meat and poultry: lean beef, ham, chicken breast, turkey breast, roast lamb or veal, and pork tenderloin
- Fish sources: salmon, tuna, trout, shrimp and scallops. Lobster, shellfish, and oysters
- Other sources: cottage cheese, milk, yogurt cheese, eggs, beans, nuts, peas, grains, and seeds

Tip #13: Prefer Grilled Food over Fried

As far as taste is concerned, it is difficult to choose the winner in the frying vs. grilling debate. However, when it comes to healthier cooking options, grilling wins hands-down. When you fry food, an excess amount of oil gets absorbed, resulting in higher calories. Grilling, on the other hand, reduces the fat content of the meat. Given that the fat tends to drop off the food during grilling, this results in much healthier and tastier meals.

Consuming fried foods in excess increases the risk of various health conditions, such as heart disease, high blood pressure, and type 2 diabetes. However, when you grill the food, it diminishes the possibility of developing such diseases. The shorter cooking time involved in grilling also ensures that you get the maximum nutritional value out of the food you eat. There is minimal loss of vitamins or moisture during grilling, and this ensures that the nutritional content of the food remains intact.

Tip #14: Drink Your Coffee Black

Don't you love sipping on hot coffee after a long day? However, cream and sugar-laden coffee only adds to your weight problems. If you are a coffee lover, drinking it black can be your best bet when it comes to staying in shape. Black coffee is not only calorie free, but it will also leave you feeling energized.

While you don't want to count on coffee as a weight loss strategy, it helps you by boosting your mood. Sipping on black coffee is always a better choice than indulging in sugary or fizzy drinks. Caffeine is known to be a mood lifter if consumed in moderate quantities. However, make sure you don't overdose on it, or it can cause various symptoms of anxiety, increased heart rate, and interrupted sleep patterns. According to the Maryland Medical Center, about two to three cups of coffee is the recommended caffeine consumption in a day. If you prefer to sip on more than three cups, choose decaf coffee.

Tip #15: Do not cut down on Carbs completely

Ask anyone you know whether there is a secret formula for weight loss, and they will quickly respond with "stop eating carbs." While cutting out carbs can certainly help you lose weight, it doesn't mean that you lose fat. This can cause some serious long-term damage to the body. Of course, if you get rid of all the pasta, bread, and potatoes from your diet, you are going to weigh much less, and if you stop eating junk food completely, the loss is going to be even greater. However, banning carbohydrates completely, including the healthier ones from vegetables and fruit, will cause you to suffer from some serious mood swings and a major drop in your energy levels.

Other side effects of completely cutting down on carbs include brain fog and dizziness. You will also experience remarkably saggy and dry skin, that could make you look 10 years older.

Why are carbs so important? Carbohydrates are the primary source of readily available energy in your body, and any deprivation can interrupt the body's functioning. Instead, be smart about your choice of carbohydrates, and balance them out with a good amount of proteins and whole foods.

Tip #16: Limit Alcohol Consumption

So you have been sweating it out at the gym. You are eating clean, watching your portion sizes, consuming less sugar, and, to top it off, you are also getting enough sleep. You aren't even partying as much, but somehow, you haven't been able to shake that one thing off your routine – and that's alcohol.

You know the feeling. Giving up on alcohol isn't that easy. Even if you decide to eliminate it, you may find yourself succumbing to peer pressure at social gatherings, and you aren't even sure whether you want to completely forego drinking alcohol.

The good news is that you can continue to drink alcohol using the right approach and still stay in shape. You don't need to go alcohol-free to achieve a great body. You can, by all means, enjoy a glass of wine after your meals. One glass of wine contains up to 150 calories, and if you can fit that into your daily calorie count, then why not?

Tip #17: Avoid Sugary Drinks

Quenching your thirst with a fizzy cola on a hot summery afternoon may feel satisfying, but it can wreak havoc on your health. There are several studies that have proven the ill effects of soda on the body. According to research, a 12-ounce serving of cola can contain about 140 calories and 39 grams of sugar. If you have been sipping on some Coke after every meal, it's time to give up this habit. Packaged milkshakes, fizzy drinks, and margaritas are not the only culprits. In fact, some of the seemingly innocent drinks can make you put on unwanted weight without you even realizing it. Even some of the healthiest sports drinks are loaded with sugar.

Did you know that consuming a sports drink right after you exercise can completely redo the calorie deficit you earned? Packaged juice is another drink that is loaded with calories. Instead, you may benefit more from actually eating your fruit instead of drinking them.

Moreover, not all fruit juices provide you with high nutritional value. Some juices with less nutritional value include pear juice, white grape juice, and apple juice. The ones with high nutritional value are cranberry juice, grape juice, vegetable juice, orange juice, and tomato juice. If at all you do prefer juicing instead of eating whole fruits, make sure you are consuming fresh juices without any added sugar.

Tip #18: Eat Your Dinner Early

We know how not getting enough sleep can make us sluggish the next day. Having an early dinner means you get to hit the sack early and, in turn, get proper sleep. Now, you can't lose weight simply because you are eating early dinners, but it helps in smoother digestion. During the night, our physical activities decrease, and hence, metabolism takes a hit, too. When you eat the last meal of the day by around 7 p.m., it leaves you with a gap of around 12 to 14 hours until you have your next day's breakfast. This gap allows your body to digest the food easily.

Tip #19: Be Patient

Don't we all wish that we had a magic wand that would make all our extra weight disappear? Just a wave of the wand, and you could instantly get washboard abs or sculpted arms. As appealing as that sounds, it may not be as rewarding as you think.

Instant gratification can discourage you from leading a healthier and much happier life. Throw a bit of patience into the game, and weight loss can be one of the most soul-satisfying journeys of your life. A few things you need to remember while watching your progress are as follows:

- Tone down that obsession: Don't weigh yourself every day. It's a sure-fire way of losing motivation. People tend to become fixated on their daily weight fluctuations and start starving or completely giving up on their goals. Instead, focus on feeling good, be consistent, and weigh yourself only towards the end of your weight loss plan.

- Break your bigger goals into smaller ones: Target a bigger goal, but be realistic. Don't jump your guns and start following it recklessly. Allow your body and mind to adapt to the changes in the diet and fitness routine. To stay motivated, make smaller goals, and reward yourself each time you achieve them.

- Be flexible: If you feel an intense rush after your workout and think you can do more, go ahead. On the other hand, if you feel exhausted after that first set of squats, go slower. Listen to your body, and don't burn yourself out.

- One of the best ways to stay patient is to keep your goals to yourself. You will find it easier to stay focused when you don't have friends or family members constantly asking you about your progress.

Tip #20: Journal Your Food Intake

Maintaining a food journal is one of the best ways to track your eating habits, including how much you eat, what foods you consume, and how it makes you feel after you eat. Getting in shape is not just about eating less or working out more, but it's also important to feel good.

When you keep a sort of a food diary, it also helps you recognize probable food intolerances or allergies, and if you aim to achieve your desired weight loss goal, tracking your daily calories through a journal is the best way.

For starters, just write down everything about your food habits for three consecutive days, or use an app to track your progress. Writing down how you feel before your meals can help you become more aware of what you eat. This can, in turn, help you to make healthier choices every time you feel tempted to indulge in unhealthy food items.

To make the most of your food journal, you have to keep track of the right things. Take a look at the five things you need to pay more attention to while food journaling.

- Pick the right method.
- Record your emotions, too.
- Be completely honest with yourself. If you do not feel good after eating a certain food item, no matter how healthy it seems, eliminate it from your meals.
- Don't fret too much about your calorie intake.
- Use your food journal to learn to know about your eating habits and how your body reacts to them.

Conclusion

Who thought getting in shape would be that easy? But here's a word of caution: if weight loss is your ultimate goal, you won't get anywhere if you miss the key ingredient, which is patience. Understand that your body is going to take some time to allow the changes to take place, so don't expect results too soon.

The actual time it takes to show results depends on how disciplined you are when it comes to following the tips given in this book. It is absolutely certain that you will feel much lighter and more energized within weeks of following the tips given in this book. You will not just lose weight but also lose your negative habits.

These nutritional tips can be life-changing if followed consistently over a period of time. We hope that in the coming days, you would obsess more about your daily nutritional intake rather than weight loss, and everything will fall into place.

Thank you, and remember to share how well these nutrition tips work for you. You can do that by writing a review in your Amazon account under Your Orders > Digital Orders.

Thank you,

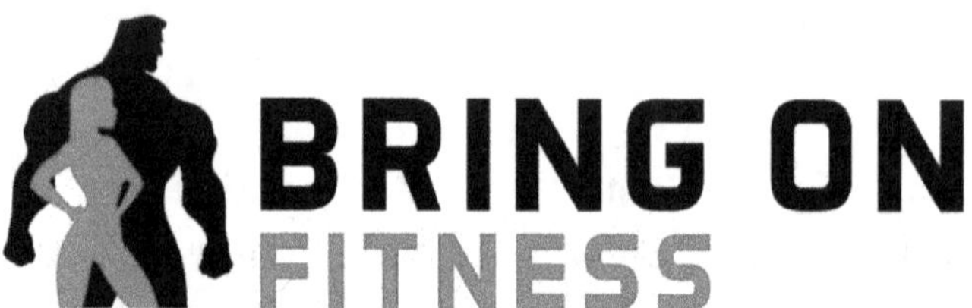

Sources

http://routineexcellence.com/fitness-motivation-tips/

http://www.health.com/weight-loss/30-simple-diet-and-fitness-tips

https://www.shape.com/lifestyle/mind-and-body/50-must-know-fitness-tips-score-your-best-body

www.ingramcontent.com/pod-product-compliance
Lightning Source LLC
Chambersburg PA
CBHW051929250726
48659CB00002B/911